Multiple Choice Questions on Lecture Notes on Clinical Medicine

Multiple Choice Questions on Lecture Notes on Clinical Medicine

DAVID RUBENSTEIN
MA MD FRCP (Lond.)
Physician
Addenbrooke's Hospital,
Cambridge

DAVID WAYNE
MA BM FRCP (Lond. & Edin.)
Physician
District Hospital
Gorleston, Great Yarmouth

SECOND EDITION

BLACKWELL SCIENTIFIC PUBLICATIONS
OXFORD LONDON EDINBURGH
BOSTON MELBOURNE

Editorial offices:
Osney Mead, Oxford OX2 0EL
8 John Street, London WC1N 2ES
9 Forrest Road, Edinburgh EH1 2QH
52 Beacon Street, Boston,
Massachusetts 02108, USA
99 Barry Street, Carlton, Victoria 3053
Australia

First published 1978
Reprinted 1979, 1980
Second edition 1982

Set by Burns & Smith, Derby
Printed and bound in
Great Britain by
Billing and Sons Ltd, Worcester

DISTRIBUTORS

USA
Blackwell Mosby Book Distributors
11830 Westline Industrial Drive
St Louis, Missouri 63141

Canada
Blackwell Mosby Book Distributors
120 Melford Drive, Scarborough
Ontario M1B 2X4

Australia
Blackwell Scientific Book Distributors
214 Berkeley Street, Carlton
Victoria 3053

British Library
Cataloguing in Publication Data

Rubenstein, David
Multiple choice questions on lecture notes on clinical medicine — 2nd ed.
1. Pathology 2.Medicine
I. Title II. Wayne, David
616 RB111

ISBN 0-632-00976-4

CONTENTS

PREFACE

The chief use of Multiple Choice Questions (MCQs) is in revision and discussion. They can sharpen a student's jaded mind — there can be no self-deceiving excuses for a wrong answer after it has been written down. Thus unrecognised lacunae in knowledge can be discovered and corrected. Accordingly, we recommend that the student answer these questions on his own by *writing out* the answers to a whole block of questions. This is preferable to looking up the answer to each question one by one after making a half-hearted mental commitment. This also avoids spoiling the next question by inadvertently spotting the answers to it. It is best to discuss the answers in groups, preferably with a tutor. The merits and de-merits of alternative answers can then be discussed and the appropriate authorities checked in case of disagreement. If you do not like the answers given in this book, you will feel more secure in your disagreement if a whole group of doctors agrees with you. If you think we have made a mistake, please write and tell us.

The case histories are included to provoke discussion of those topics which we feel benefit most from this approach. The answers given are a brief guide for those who are working on their own. They may help to generate some steam in group discussions — we do not claim that they are the only possible answers.

In this Second edition, we have modified many questions, corrected some answers and added new questions on poisoning and diseases of travellers.

Reading textbooks is generally very boring and we hope that these questions will add a hint of enjoyment to the grind of study. Good luck — we hope you get all of them right.

May 1982

David Rubenstein
David Wayne

PART ONE

1. Bitemporal hemianopia can occur with:

A Temporal lobe astrocytoma
B Craniopharyngioma
C Pinealoma
D Internal carotid aneurysm
E Pituitary tumour

2. Sudden blindness occurs with:

A Vitreous haemorrhage
B Choroido-retinitis of toxoplasmosis
C Temporal arteritis
D Glaucoma
E Neurosyphilis

3. A small pupil is seen in:

A Argyll Robertson pupil
B Third nerve palsy
C Holmes-Adie syndrome
D Meiotic drugs
E Mydriatic drugs

4. The following are typical of Horner's syndrome:

A Enophthalmos
B Anhydrosis
C Pupillary dilatation
D Ptosis

5. Which of the following muscle innervations are correct:

A Biceps: C 3–4
B Triceps: C 7
C Iliopsoas: L 23
D Sternomastoid: C 1–2
E Deltoid in shoulder abduction: C 4–5

6. Which of the following reflex innervations are correct:

A Knee jerk: L 3–4
B Ankle jerk: L 5
C Triceps jerk: C 6
D Biceps jerk: C 5–6
E Supinator jerk: C 7

7. Which two of the following are the more common causes of paraesthesiae in the fingers:

A Multiple sclerosis
B Cervical rib
C Cervical spondylosis
D Carpal tunnel syndrome
E Vitamin B_{12} deficiency

8. Carpal tunnel syndrome occurs in:

A Syringomyelia
B Pregnancy
C Myxoedema
D Rheumatoid arthritis
E Gout
F The contraceptive pill

9. **Ulnar nerve lesions are characterised by:**
A Weakness of all thenar muscles
B Weakness of all the hypothenar muscles
C Wrist drop
D Sensory loss over thumb, index and middle fingers
E Sensory loss over ring and little fingers

10. **Ptosis:**
A May follow a partial 7th nerve lesion
B Occurs in myotonia congenita
C Occurs in myasthenia gravis
D Is partial in lesions of the sympathetic nerves
E May be congenital

11. **Facial nerve palsy:**
A Movements of the forehead are retained if the upper motor neurone is involved
B Is an early feature of acoustic neuroma
C Occurs in sarcoid
D Occurs in Guillain–Barré syndrome
E Occurs in poliomyelitis
F Is associated with herpes zoster infection

12. **Which of the following are true:**
A Pain and temperature tracts are ipsilateral to the dermatomes
B Vibration sense is carried in the dorsal columns
C Patients veer away from the side of cerebellar lesions
D Dissociated anaesthesia is a feature of motor neurone disease
E The tremor of Parkinson's disease improves on movement

13. The following are features of hypermetropia:

A Concave spectacle lenses
B Short sightedness
C Small optic disc on ophthalmoscopy
D Temporal pallor of the disc
E Absent ankle and sometimes knee jerks

14. Subacute combined degeneration of the cord is associated with:

A Damage to the dorso-lateral columns
B MCV of more than $90\mu^3$
C Absent knee jerks
D Brisk ankle jerks
E Diminished sensation to all modalities

15. Posterior uveitis is associated with:

A Inflammation of the choroid
B Diabetes mellitus
C Diabetes insipidus
D Sarcoidosis with normal calcium
E Sarcoidosis with high calcium
F Toxoplasmosis

16. Xanthelasma and xanthelasma-like lesions occur in:

A Hyperthyroidism
B Diabetes mellitus
C Pseudoxanthoma elasticum
D Primary biliary cirrhosis
E Hypercholesterolaemia
F Dermatomyositis

17. Cataracts are associated with:

A Rubella
B Hyperparathyroidism
C Dystrophia myotonica
D Chloramphenicol
E Diabetes mellitus
F Hypothyroidism
G Chloroquine

18. Very large spleens are typically found with:

A Infectious hepatitis
B Pernicious anaemia
C Myelofibrosis
D Chronic myeloid leukaemia
E Long standing cirrhosis

19. In which of the following is ascites usually present on clinical examination:

A Left ventricular failure
B Cirrhosis of the liver
C Intra-abdominal Hodgkin's disease
D Nephrotic syndrome
E Carcinoma of the uterus

20. Unconjugated hyperbilirubinaemia is characteristic of:

A Gilbert's syndrome
B Dubin–Johnson syndrome
C Rotor syndrome
D Haemolytic anaemia
E Chronic active hepatitis

21. Jaundice with pale stools and dark urine is characteristic of:

A Infectious hepatitis
B Carcinoma of the pancreas
C Hepatoma
D Glandular fever hepatitis
E Primary biliary cirrhosis
F Chlorpromazine jaundice

22. In obstructive jaundice of the elderly the following may help distinguish between the causes:

A Bilirubin level
B Alkaline phosphatase
C α-feto-protein
D Serum albumin
E Prothrombin time
F Mitochondrial antibody estimation

23. Which of the following may cause dysphagia:

A Achalasia of the cardia
B Motor neurone disease
C Myasthenia gravis
D Parkinson's disease
E Syringomyelia
F Carcinoma of the stomach

24. The following are typical presenting features of achalasia of the cardia:

A Mediastinal widening on chest X-ray
B Retrosternal pain with acid regurgitation
C Recurrent pneumonia
D Dysphagia initially with solids more than liquids
E Weight loss

25. **Diarrhoea may occur with:**

A Pernicious anaemia
B Diabetes mellitus
C Sarcoidosis
D Lincomycin
E Thyrotoxicosis
F Carcinoid syndrome

26. **Which of the following are likely to cause acute abdominal pain and rectal bleeding in the elderly:**

A Haemorrhoids
B Ischaemic colitis
C Diverticular disease
D Ulcerative colitis
E Carcinoma of the colon
F Carcinoma of the head of the pancreas

27. **Haemoptysis occurs characteristically in the following:**

A Tuberculosis
B Pulmonary sarcoidosis
C Mitral stenosis
D Bronchial adenoma
E Polyarteritis nodosa
F Bronchiectasis

28. **The following characterise fibrosing alveolitis:**

A Low FEV/FVC ratio
B Normal FEV/FVC ratio
C High $PaCO_2$
D Low $PaCO_2$
E Low PaO_2

29. Central cyanosis characteristically occurs with:

A Over 5 g/100 ml reduced haemoglobin
B Pulmonary aspergillosis
C Status asthmaticus
D Congenital pulmonary stenosis
E Polycythaemia rubra vera
F Multiple pulmonary emboli

30. In chronic cor pulmonale the following signs are characteristic:

A Immediate blowing diastolic pulmonary murmur
B Quiet pulmonary second sound
C Left parasternal diffuse heave
D Hepatomegaly
E Large 'v' wave in JVP

31. Methaemoglobinaemia is caused by:

A Aspirin
B Phenacetin
C Phenylbutazone
D Shoe polish
E Primaquine
F Clindamycin

32. The following commonly occur in left ventricular failure:

A Paroxysmal nocturnal dyspnoea
B Fine bilateral basal crepitations
C Right-sided pleural effusion
D Reversed splitting of the second sound
E Splenomegaly
F Pansystolic murmur at the apex

33. Reduced arterial pulse volume (and pressure) are found in:

A Atrial septal defect
B Pulmonary stenosis
C Mitral stenosis
D Patent ductus arteriosus
E Pericardial tamponade

34. Increased pulse volume occurs in:

A Syphylitic aortic incompetence
B Rheumatic mitral incompetence
C Mitral incompetence immediately following myocardial infarction
D Atrial septal defect
E Paget's disease

35. Atrial fibrillation is a typical feature of:

A Ischaemic heart disease
B Friedreich's ataxia
C Amyloid
D Thyrotoxicosis
E Mitral stenosis
F Constrictive pericarditis

36. A prominent 'a' wave may suggest:

A Atrial flutter with changing block
B Tricuspid incompetence
C Ventricular septal defect
D Pulmonary stenosis
E Pulmonary hypertension
F Complete heart block

37. A prominent 'v' wave may suggest:

A Atrial flutter with changing block
B Tricuspid incompetence
C Ventricular septal defect
D Pulmonary stenosis
E Pulmonary hypertension
F Complete heart block

38. The following are typical of mitral stenosis:

A Mid-diastolic rumbling murmur
B Opening snap just following the first sound
C Loud first sound
D Recurrent chest infection
E Relative reduction in blood flow to apices of the lung

39. In aortic coarctation:

A Patients are always under 40 at presentation
B Cyanosis may result if untreated
C The murmur may best be heard between the scapulae
D Radio-femoral delay is associated with scapular anastomosis
E Hypertension is invariably reversed by surgery

40. In rheumatic aortic stenosis

A The pulse volume is reduced
B There is a pansystolic apical murmur
C The aortic second sound is 'clicking' in character
D There is a thrill at the base of the heart

41. In sub-valvar aortic stenosis:

A The arterial pulse character is 'slow rise and fall'
B The murmur radiates to the neck
C The aortic second sound is normal
D β-blocking agents may be helpful

42. In the ECG:

A Left axis deviation may occur in right bundle branch block
B The upper limit of the QRS complex is 0.12 sec
C The 'p' mitrale is best seen in the central chest leads
D The PR interval varies normally with heart rate
E Left bundle branch block is not usually pathological

43. The following are true:

A Delta waves occur in hypothyroidism
B 'U' waves are seen in hypokalaemia
C The 'T' waves are peaked in hyperkalaemia
D 'J' waves suggest hypocalcaemia
E Digitalis toxicity causes ST elevation
F The QT interval is increased in hypercalcaemia

44. The following are useful in the treatment of acute pulmonary oedema:

A Posture
B Oxygen
C Frusemide
D β_2 stimulants
E β_1 blockers
F Aminophylline
G Heroin

PART TWO

NEUROLOGY

45. Cluster headaches:

A Suggest the presence of an underlying tumour
B Are rarely unilateral
C Typically cause unilateral congestion of the eye and nostril
D Are sometimes precipited by phenylbutazone
E Usually respond to ergotamine

46. The following features are characteristic of trigeminal neuralgia:

A Onset usually between 30 and 40 years
B Rarely unilateral
C Sulthiame is a drug of first choice
D Relieved sometimes by carbamazepine
E Triggered by chewing
F An auditory aura may precede attack

47. Subdural haematoma:

A Is more common in the elderly alcoholic
B May be present with progressive dementia
C A history of previous trauma is invariable
D Ipsilateral headache often indicates the side of the lesion
E May be bilateral

48. Extradural haematoma:

A A history of previous trauma is invariable
B The patient is usually over 40
C Presenile dementia may be the presenting feature
D Loss of consciousness is uncommon
E Loss of consciousness is a late event

49. Which of the following occur in the lateral medullary syndrome (posterior inferior cerebellar artery thrombosis):

A Dysphagia
B Ipsilateral Horner's syndrome
C Nystagmus to the side of the lesion
D Ipsilateral cerebellar signs
E Ipsilateral 5th nerve dissociated sensory deficit
F Contralateral dissociated anaesthesia to the limbs

50. Which of the following features will help distinguish between grand mal epilepsy and other causes of transient unconsciousness in the elderly:

A The presence of an aura
B Aortic stenosis
C A history of chronic bronchitis
D Right bundle branch block on the ECG
E Perspiration with attacks

51. Petit mal:

A Usually begins in early adolescence
B Is characterised by tongue biting during attacks
C Is commonly associated with migraine
D Has characteristic EEG with spike and wave formation at 30 cycles per second
E Attacks may be followed by automatism

52. **Meningitis:**

A Is usually caused by enteroviruses
B The meningococcus and *Haemophilus influenzae* are the common bacteria in adult meningitis
C Penicillin is the treatment of choice for pneumococcal and *Haemophilus influenzae* meningitis
D Meningococci appear as Gram-positive diplococci
E *Leptospira icterohaemorrhagica* may cause meningitis and is sensitive to penicillin

53. **Multiple sclerosis is suggested by:**

A Transient diplopia in a 24-year old woman
B Pain in eye, blurring of vision in a 74-year old man
C Slow progressive paraplegia in a 60-year old woman
D Trigeminal neuralgia in a 30-year old woman
E Bilateral blurring of near vision, 40-year old woman

54. **Extrapyramidal symptoms may be caused by:**

A Levodopa
B Chlorpromazine in the absence of jaundice
C Copper deposition in the CNS
D Haloperidol
E Chloramphenicol
F Primaquine
G Reserpine

55. **Patients with Parkinson's disease may improve with:**

A Atropine
B Levodopa
C Ethosuximide
D Methysergide
E Benzhexol
F Amantidine
G Amitryptiline if the patient is depressed
H Bromocryptine

56. **The following are features of Wilson's disease:**

A Kayser-Fleischer rings which are diagnostic and due to copper deposition
B Inheritance is recessive
C High copper levels in serum
D Increased serum caeruloplasmin levels
E Slurred speech
F Normal urinary copper

57. **Huntington's chorea:**

A Is transmitted as a Mendelian recessive
B Characteristically first presents in late teens and early 20's
C Affects mainly the limbs and face
D Is improved by levodopa
E Is improved by tetrabenazine
F Progressive dementia is common

58. **Raised intracranial pressure is suggested by:**

A Photophobia
B Blurring of vision
C Neck stiffness and positive Kernig's sign
D Headache characteristically present on waking
E Nausea

59. **Acoustic neuromas:**

A Are fibromas of the 7th cranial nerve and thereby cause facial palsy
B Are bilateral in 30% of cases
C May cause tinnitus and deafness
D May cause vertigo
E Do not usually alter the CSF

60. Edrophonium:

A Rapidly reverses muscle fatigue in myasthenia gravis
B Rapidly reverses muscle fatigue in Eaton-Lambert syndrome
C Inhibits cholinesterase
D Is reversed rapidly by pyridostigmine
E Is effective orally only if given not less than 6-hourly

61. The following features of motor neurone disease are characteristic:

A Onset normally between 15 and 25
B Upper motor neurone destruction is uncommon
C Diminution of sensation to light touch and pain with loss of reflexes
D Neostigmine rarely gives improvement
E Life expectancy is 10–15 years after presentation

62. In Friedreich's ataxia:

A Death may occur from heart failure
B Absent reflexes in the legs may be associated with up-going plantar responses
C Dementia is a common early finding
D Cerebellar ataxia is a common early finding
E Bulbar palsy is a late feature

63. The following are typical features of tabes dorsalis as compared with meningo-vascular syphilis:

A Lightning pains
B Onset within 5–10 years of original infection
C Ptosis
D Sensory deficit over the nose and sternum
E Transverse myelitis and paraplegia

64. Poliomyelitis can be distinguished from Guillain-Barré syndrome by

A Growing a RNA virus from the CSF and stools
B Paralysis is virtually always preceded by meningitis
C Paralysis of the limbs is symmetrical in poliomyelitis
D Very high CSF protein (over 50 g/l)
E The complete absence of sensory changes

65. Syringomyelia causes:

A Sensory deficit to pain and vibration in the hands
B Wasting of the small hand muscles
C Horner's syndrome
and may be improved by:
D Vitamin B_{12} injections
E Neurosurgery

66. In a patient with a sudden onset of weakness in both legs:

A Hysteria is the most common cause
B Subacute combined degeneration is a likely cause
C If a young man he may have prolapsed a disc
D Lumbar puncture should be performed urgently
E A neurological opinion must be sought as an emergency

PSYCHIATRY

67. In depression:

A Paranoid delusions are common
B Early morning waking is characteristic
C There is loss of libido
D Memory for recent events is poor
E Tricyclic antidepressants have adrenergic side effects

68. The following are well recognised causes of acute confusion:

A Acute porphyria
B Thyrotoxicosis
C Myxoedema
D Hypoglycaemia
E Cushing's syndrome

69. Elderly patients with dementia:

A Lose memory for recent more than past events
B Suffer from marked emotional lability
C Have paranoid delusions
D Typically lose interest in friends and relatives
E Are frequently depressed
F May occasionally respond to vitamin B_{12} or thyroxine

70. Schizophrenia:

A Occurs in about 0.5% of the population
B Eventually always requires hospitalisation despite phenothiazine therapy
C May be familial
D Is frequently associated with shyness and hallucinations

CONNECTIVE TISSUE AND RHEUMATIC DISEASES

71. Polyarteritis nodosa:

A May present with myocardial infarction
B Is associated with LE cells in 80% of cases
C Hypertension occurs in 60% of cases
D Presents as late onset asthma in 20% of cases
E Abdominal pain occurs in 25% of cases
F Renal failure is uncommon

72. Dermatomyositis is characterised by:

A Onset at 23–35, mainly in women
B Underlying malignancy
C Cardiac failure
D Telangiectasia affecting mainly the face and upper chest
E Occasionally improves with prednisolone despite chronicity

73. Systemic sclerosis may result in:

A Malabsorption
B Renal failure
C Presenile dementia
D Pulmonary fibrosis
E Mononeuritis multiplex

74. The following features typify polymalgia rheumatica:

A Weakness of proximal upper limb muscles
B Onset usually between 50 and 60
C Underlying carcinoma
D ESR raised between 50 and 70
E Slow but progressive response to steroids

75. Which of the following are features of systemic lupus erythematosus:

A Thrombocytopenia
B Fits
C Pericardial friction rub
D Plate-like atelectasis on chest X-ray
E Isolated pleural effusion

76. Temporal arteritis is associated with:

A Headache usually severe and always unilateral
B ESR of about 100
C Pyrexia which may be the presenting symptom
D Sudden blindness
and is
E usually excluded by a normal temporal artery biopsy

77. The following complicate or occur with rheumatoid arthritis:

A Acanthosis nigricans
B Episcleritis
C Malabsorption
D Carpal tunnel syndrome
E Amyloid
F Retinitis pigmentosa

78. Which of the following are true of rheumatoid arthritis:

A Severe disability occurs in 25–30%
B Amyloid is rare but usually a serious complication
C Chloroquine is sometimes useful but may cause cataract
D Splenomegaly occurs in about 15% of patients
E Joint involvement is usually asymmetrical
F Lung involvement is rarely important

79. Rheumatoid factor is:

A A circulating IgM immunoglobulin
B Usually present if subcutaneous nodules are present
C Positive in over 85% of patients with rheumatoid arthritis
D Usually present in psoriatic arthritis
E Usually present in ankylosing spondylitis
F Present in some healthy people

80. Felty's syndrome is characterised by:

A Involvement of large joints
B Lymphadenopathy
C Hypersplenism
D Improvement of joint symptoms following splenectomy
E Positive rheumatoid factor

81. In Sjögren's syndrome the following are usually true:

A Negative rheumatoid factor
B Vaginal atrophy
C Positive Schirmer's test
D Positive antinuclear factor
E Xerostomia

82. The following are features of psoriatic arthritis:

A Subcutaneous nodules
B Negative rheumatoid factor
C Severe mutilating arthritis
D Involvement of the distal interphalangeal joints
E Associated sacroileitis

83. Joint involvement is characteristically symmetrical in:

A Osteoarthritis
B Gonococcal arthritis
C Rheumatoid arthritis
D Gout
E Psoriatic arthritis

84. In ankylosing spondylitis:

A Ulcerative colitis may coexist
B Iritis occurs in 30%
C Rheumatoid factor is usually present
D Respiratory failure may occur
E There is high correlation with HLA 13

85. Reiter's disease is associated with:

A Sacroileitis
B Muscular spasm (Reiter's cramp)
C Pustular hyperkeratosis of the palms
D Circinate balanitis
E Bacillary dysentery
F Positive Reiter's complement fixation test (about 60%)

ENDOCRINE DISEASE

86. Acromegaly is associated with:

A Bitemporal upper quadrantic hemianopia
B Thickening of the heel pad and tufting of the terminal phalanges
C Raised levels of growth hormone which can be suppressed with glucose
D Hypertension in about a quarter of patients
E Excessive perspiration

87. Polyuria and polydipsia occur in:

A Acute glomerulonephritis
B Hysterical polydipsia
C Hyperkalaemia
D Hypocalcaemia
E Intracranial sarcoid

88. Which of the following occur in hyperthyroidism:

A Raised TSH levels
B Vitiligo
C Atrial fibrillation which is reversed by digitalis
D Tachycardia which is sensitive to β-blockade
E Carpal tunnel syndrome

89. Which of the following may be related to hypothyroidism:

A Congenital blindness
B Low serum B_{12}
C Low serum folate
D Congenital deafness
E 'J' waves on the ECG
F Psoriasis

90. Thyroid enlargement may occur with:

A Hashimoto's disease
B Aspirin therapy
C Phenacetin therapy
D Carbimazole therapy
E Phenylbutazone therapy

91. Which of the following are true:

A The TRH test is helpful in secondary hypothyroidism
B Anaemia in myxoedema may be macrocytic
C TSH is reduced in primary hypothyroidism
D β-blockade is adequate therapy in mild hyperthyroidism
E Iodine uptake is reduced by PAS, INAH and propylthiouracil

92. Thyroid carcinoma:

A Usually takes up excessive radioactive iodine
B Is usually 'Follicular' and may present as an enlarged gland in the neck
C Sometimes regresses if thyroxine is given
D Follows radiation to the neck
E May secrete parathormone

93. The following complicate steroid therapy:

A Vitiligo
B Diabetes mellitus
C Anhydrosis
D Diabetes insipidus
E Osteoporosis
F Hypercalcaemia
G Skin atrophy

94. In Cushing's syndrome:

A Adrenal adenomas are present in 20%
B Adrenal carcinomas are present in 10%
C Hyperpigmentation is found in the buccal mucosa
D Confusion may occur
E Proximal myopathy may occur
F The diurnal cortisol variation is exaggerated

95. The Waterhouse Friderichsen syndrome is characterised by:

A Paroxysmal hypertension
B Generalised purpura
C Pneumococcal septicaemia
D Acute adrenal haemorrhage

96. Phaeochromocytoma:

A Usually presents with paroxysmal hypertension
B Is invariably benign
C May not always be found in the adrenal gland
D Is easily detected on IVP
E May be detected by ultrasound

97. In carcinoid syndrome:

A The primary tumour is usually in the ileum
B Liver metastases are invariably present
C Asthma and/or diarrhoea may occur
D Pulmonary stenosis occurs rarely
E Urinary VMA is raised in 70–80%

98. Which of the following are true:

A Phaeochromocytomas cause α and β adrenergic effects
B Bronchial adenomas are usually carcinoid tumours
C Conn's syndrome results from adenomas of the zona fasciculata
D Growth hormone deficiency is never an isolated phenomenon
E The Synacthen (tetracosactrin test) may help distinguish adrenal hyperplasia from carcinoma

METABOLIC DISEASE

99. Diabetes mellitus is present if:

A The fasting sugar is 6.7 mmol/l (120 mg/dl)
B A random sugar is 8.9 mmol/l (160 mg/dl)
C 2-hour post-prandial sugar is 11 mmol/l (200 mg/dl)
D Microaneurysms are present
E Nodular glomerular sclerosis is present

100. The following complications definitely improve with good diabetic control:

A Peripheral neuropathy
B Mononeuritis multiplex
C Vulvo-vaginitis
D Proximal amyotrophy (Garland's syndrome)
E Angina
F Lipodystrophy

101. Glycosuria may occur with:

A Phaeochromocytoma
B Carcinoid tumour
C Cushing's syndrome
D Haemochromatosis
E Subarachnoid haemorrhage
F Hepato-lenticular degeneration

102. Which of the following kidney disorders occur in diabetes mellitus:

A Diffuse glomerular sclerosis
B Nodular glomerular sclerosis
C Pyelonephritis
D Acute papillary necrosis
E Nephrotic syndrome

103. In diabetes mellitus which of the following may occur:

A Retinitis proliferans
B Retinitis pigmentosa
C Necrobiosis lipoidica
D Nocturnal diarrhoea

104. In diabetic ketoacidosis:

A Underlying infection is invariably present
B Previous diabetes is unsuspected in 60%
C Gastric dilatation is common and may lead to aspiration pneumonia
D Fluid replacement may cause considerable improvement before insulin is started
E Long-term insulin will always be needed

105. Which of the following are true:

A Lactic acidosis tends to occur in insulin dependent diabetes
B Hyperosmolar coma is more common in the elderly and obese
C Large doses of insulin are usually required in diabetic lactic acidosis
D Large doses of insulin are required in hyperosmolar coma
E Ketonuria is minimal in lactic acidosis and hyperosmolar coma

106. In acute intermittent porphyria:

A Abdominal pain may be the presenting symptom
B Hypotension and bradycardia are characteristic
C Photosensitivity is common
D Urinary porphobilinogen is raised and makes the urine darken on standing in the light

107. In Type IV hyperlipidaemia:

A The triglycerides are predominantly raised
B The chylomicrons are predominantly raised
C Diabetes and gout may be associated
D Achilles tendinitis may be associated
E Nephrotic syndrome may be the presenting feature

108. In osteoporosis:

A Bone fractures are uncommon
B Proximal myopathy occurs
C The bone matrix is calcified normally
D Underlying thyrotoxicosis may be present
E Oestrogen therapy is effective

109. Tetanus may occur with or following:

A Radio-iodine therapy
B *Clostridium welchii* infection
C Osteomalacia
D Hyperventilation syndrome
E Partial thyroidectomy

110. Which of the following are true:

A 1-25-Hydroxycholecalciferol is made in the liver
B Sclerotic deposits occur rarely in myeloma
C The alkaline phosphatase is elevated in osteoporosis
D The alkaline phosphatase is greatly elevated in Paget's disease
E Salmon calcitonin may relieve bone pain in Paget's disease

111. Hyperparathyroidism may be complicated by:

A Psychosis
B Peptic ulceration
C Renal colic
D Thirst, vomiting and constipation
E Proximal myopathy

112. Hypercalcaemia is caused by:

A Hypervitaminosis D
B Oat cell carcinoma of the lung
C Sarcoid
D Multiple myelomatosis
E Pseudo-pseudohypoparathyroidism
F Secondary hyperparathyroidism
G Tertiary hyperparathyroidism

113. Hypercalcaemic patients may respond to:

A Aluminium hydroxide
B Intravenous saline
C Intravenous phosphate
D Bendrofluazide
E Corticosteroids
F Oral methyl-testosterone
G Intramuscular calcitonin
H Bed rest and immobilisation

114. Acute gout may be caused by:

A Aspirin
B Indomethacin
C Allopurinol
D Bendrofluazide
E Phenylbutazone
F Treatment of Hodgkin's disease

115. Gout is associated with:

A Hyperthyroidism
B Hypertension
C Negative refractile crystals in joint fluid
D Pseudocyst formation on X-ray in the periarticular regions
E Renal colic

116. Which of the following may be useful in acute gout:

A Allopurinol
B Phenylbutazone
C Aspirin
D Indomethacin
E Pyrazinamide

117. Calcification of cartilage occurs in:

A Osteopetrosis
B Hyperparathyroidism
C Pseudo-gout
D Chronic osteoarthritis
E Reiter's disease

RENAL DISEASE

118. On the IVP:

A Normal adult kidneys are about 10 cm in length
B 'Fetal lobulation' is associated with intrinsic disease
C Excretion of dye is normally complete in 20–30 minutes
D Polycystic disease produces a characteristic appearance
E Acute tubular necrosis produces a diagnostic appearance

119. Polyuria and polydipsia may be presenting features of:

A Hyperkalaemia
B Chronic glomerular nephritis
C Nephrogenic diabetes insipidus
D Hypocalcaemia
E Diabetes mellitus

120. In the nephrotic syndrome:

A Underlying diabetes mellitus is present in about 50%
B The blood urea may be low, normal or high
C Peripheral oedema is not always present
D Proteinuria is rarely less than 8–10 g/24 hours
E Microscopic haematuria is invariably present

121. In acute tubular necrosis

A The patient is invariably symptomatically very ill
B Hypotension is present
C Hypotension may be the cause
D Urine output is less than 400 ml/24 hours

122. The following are typical features of chronic renal failure

A Anaemia
B Raised serum calcium
C Raised serum phosphate
D Raised serum bicarbonate
E Urine specific gravity is high

123. Which of the following are true:

A Urine specific gravity in hypovolaemia is high
B Urine specific gravity in tubular necrosis is high
C Phenacetin and primaquine cause analgesic nephropathy
D Gentamicin (given alone) is nephrotoxic
E Uraemic bone disease may be helped by 1-α-hydroxycholecalciferol

124. Which of the following are true:

A Serum complement is reduced in chronic glomerular nephritis

B In acute glomerular nephritis complete recovery occurs in 90% of adults and children

C Minimal change nephritis correlates with selective proteinuria and good prognosis

D Membranous change nephritis indicates good prognosis

E *E. coli* (40%) and *Proteus vulgaris* (30%) account for most urinary tract infection in general practice

125. Which of the following occur with inappropriate ADH secretion:

A Confusion and coma

B Carcinoma of the bronchus

C Progressive uraemia

D Low serum sodium with reduced osmolality

E Low urinary sodium and osmolality

126. Which of the following usually require potassium supplements:

A Bendrofluazide

B Frusemide

C Prednisolone in treatment of Addison's disease

D Cotrimoxazole

E Amiloride

127. Hypokalaemia may follow treatment with:

A Colchicine

B Triamterene

C Oxyphenbutazone

D Carbenoxolone

E Cimetidine

F Hydroxocobalamine for pernicious anaemia

128. Which of the following are true:

A Heparin is given for haemolytic uraemic syndrome
B Warfarin is given for haemolytic uraemic syndrome
C Mannitol may prevent the hepato-renal syndrome
D Prostatectomy may induce sodium retention
E 60% of body weight is water

LIVER DISEASE

129. Which of the following will distinguish between short and long incubation hepatitis:

A Splenomegaly
B Australia antigen (hepatitis associated antigen)
C History of alcohol
D Recent dental extraction
E Speed of recovery

130. Which of the following are true:

A Bed rest improves prognosis in serum hepatatis
B Australia antigen can be spread venereally
C γ-globulin does not protect contacts of short incubation hepatitis
D Pale stools and dark urine are early features of infectious hepatitis
E Chronic aggressive hepatitis is associated with antibodies to smóoth muscle and mitochondria and the Australia antigen

131. Porto-systemic encephalopathy may be improved by:

A Lactulose
B Pyridostigmine
C High glucose intake
D Magnesium sulphate enemas
E Neomycin

132. Liver failure may be induced by:

A Barbiturates
B Morphine
C Diazepam
D High protein diet
E High glucose diet
F Gastrointestinal haemorrhage

133. Haematemesis and melaena in a patient with cirrhosis is likely to come from:

A Bleeding oesophageal varices
B Duodenal ulceration
C Gastric ulceration
D Abnormal clotting mechanisms
E Haemorrhoids
F Hepatoma
G Carcinoma of bile duct

134. Ascites:

A Is due to portal hypertension alone (in cirrhosis)
B Sometimes responds to bed rest
C Is associated with secondary hyperaldosteronism
D Is associated with inappropriate ADH secretion
E Can be detected radiologically
F May be the presenting feature of constrictive pericarditis

135. Haemochromatosis:

A Is transmitted by a recessive gene
B Is best treated by venesection
C Is best treated with desferrioxamine
D Predisposes to chronic active hepatitis
E Predisposes to hepatoma
F Is associated with a high iron binding capacity which is fully saturated

136. Which of the following are true:

A Rosette formation on histology is typical of chronic active but not chronic persistent hepatitis
B Schistosomiasis causes cirrhosis
C Cardiac cirrhosis is characterised by nodular hyperplasia
D Hepatocellular failure may follow phenacetin poisoning
E Halothane jaundice occurs 1-2 weeks after first exposure

137. Cholestatic jaundice may result from therapy with:

A Erythromycin stearate
B Nitrofurantoin
C Chlorpromazine
D Lincomycin
E Clindamycin
F Primaquine
G Testosterone proprionate
H Phenacetin

138. Haemolytic jaundice may result from therapy with:

A Erythromycin stearate
B Nitrofurantoin
C Chlorpromazine
D Methyldopa
E Primaquine
F Testosterone proprionate
G Phenacetin

139. Gluten sensitive enteropathy:

- **A** May present in middle age
- **B** Occurs in families
- **C** Is associated with erythema annulare
- **D** Is associated with pemphigus vulgaris
- **E** Is associated with dermatitis herpetiformis
- **F** Is associated with psoriasis
- **G** Is associated with small bowel lymphoma

140. Which of the following are true:

- **A** Flocculation of barium is the cardinal feature of steatorrhea
- **B** The degree of villous atrophy in gluten sensitivity correlates approximately with prognosis
- **C** Tropical sprue is caused by *Giardia lamblia*
- **D** Normal faecal fat excretion is up to 3 g/day
- **E** Lactase deficiency responds to withdrawal of milk from the diet

141. Which of the following occur with ulcerative colitis:

- **A** Erythema nodosum
- **B** Anterior uveitis
- **C** Arthritis affecting the ankles
- **D** Colonic dilatation
- **E** Rose thorn ulcers on barium enema

142. Of the following which are the two most common hepatic complications of ulcerative colitis:

- **A** Pericholangitis
- **B** Chronic aggressive hepatitis
- **C** Carcinoma of the bile duct
- **D** Sclerosing cholangitis
- **E** Fatty infiltration

143. In ulcerative colitis:

A Oral ulceration may occur
B Salazopyrine reduces relapse rate
C A typical cobblestone appearance is seen on X-ray
D Ankylosing spondylitis occurs more commonly
E Prednisolone in large doses is required to prevent relapses
F The rectum is involved in 90% of patients

144. Which of the following are associated more with Crohn's disease than ulcerative colitis:

A Skip lesions on barium meal
B Involvement of the colonic mucosa
C Perianal inflammation
D Acute toxic dilation of the ileum
E Abdominal pain
F Stricture formation

145. Which of the following definitely accelerate healing of gastric ulcers:

A Antacids in gel form
B Bed rest at home
C Bed rest in hospital
D Stopping smoking
E Losing weight
F Stopping alcohol
G Sodium carbenoxalone (Biogastrone)
H H_2 receptor blockade

146. Which statements are true:

A Bleeding from colonic diverticula may be catastrophic
B About half of haematemeses are from gastric ulcers
C The most common cause of rectal bleeding is carcinoma of the colon
D A blood urea of 140 mg% (23 mmol/litre) following haematemesis denotes previous renal disease
E Ischaemic colitis involves mainly the hepatic flexure and transverse colon
F Whipple's disease is characterised by typical granulomas seen on jejunal biopsy

147. In the Zollinger–Ellison syndrome:

A Recurrent gastric ulceration typically occurs
B A pancreatic gastrin secreting adenoma is usually present
C The volume of gastric juice is increased to 3–4 litres/day
D The tumour is malignant in over 50% of cases
E There may be adenomas in other endocrine glands

RESPIRATORY DISEASE

148. The following are features of chronic bronchitis:

A FEV/FVC ratio often less than 60%
B Productive cough for 1 month for 2 consecutive years
C Improves on stopping smoking
D Mucolytic agents improve respiratory function
E α_1-antitrypsin deficiency
F The chest X-ray is rarely normal

149. In status asthmaticus which of the following are true:

A Corticosteroids in very large doses may cause increase in airways obstruction
B β_2 stimulant drugs may be effective
C $PaCO_2$ may be reduced
D $PaCO_2$ may be raised
E PaO_2 may be reduced
F Disodium cromoglycate should be given in high doses
G Sedation is potentially lethal

150. Which of the following are typically complicated by lung abscess formation:

A *Mycoplasma pneumoniae* infection
B Klebsiella pneumonia
C Pulmonary embolism
D Staphylococcal pneumonia
E *Haemophilus influenzae* pneumonia
F Pneumothorax

151. Which of the following usually contraindicate surgical resection of bronchial carcinoma:

A FEV of less than 1 litre
B Raised diaphragm with paradoxical movement
C Metastases
D Hoarseness of the voice
E Multiple haemoptyses
F Ectopic ACTH secretion

152. Bronchial carcinoma may be complicated by:

A Cerebellar atrophy
B Megaloblastic anaemia
C Achilles tendinitis
D ADH secretion usually from squamous cell carcinomas
E Hypercalcaemia without bone secondary deposits
F Pulmonary osteoarthropathy
G Keratoderma blenorrhagica

153. In sarcoid which of the following occur:

- **A** Erythema marginatum
- **B** Hypercalcaemia which responds to steroids
- **C** Subperiostial erosion of phalanges
- **D** Diabetes mellitus
- **E** Diabetes insipidus

154. Which of the following statements are correct:

- **A** The hepatitis of rifampicin is usually mild
- **B** Ethionamide causes visual field defects
- **C** Ethambutol is hepatotoxic
- **D** INAH peripheral neuropathy may be reversed by Vitamin B_6
- **E** Streptomycin causes deafness if renal function is poor
- **F** Streptomycin is nephrotoxic

155. Episodic dyspnoea in a young woman of 30 years is more likely to be due to pulmonary embolism if:

- **A** She takes the pill
- **B** Gallop rhythm is present on examination
- **C** She has fainting episodes with the attacks

and is unlikely if:

- **D** There are no abnormal chest signs
- **E** The chest X-ray is normal
- **F** Blood gases are normal between attacks

156. Patients with a spontaneous pneumothorax usually:

- **A** Are overweight
- **B** Have severe dyspnoea at the onset
- **C** Have severe pain at the onset
- **D** Show increased movement of the chest on the affected side
- **E** Require intercostal drainage if more than 20% of the total lung field is collapsed
- **F** Improve spontaneously with resorption of the pneumothorax

157. Which of the following are features of cryptogenic fibrosing alveolitis:

A Clubbing
B Patchy fibrosis sometimes with tracheal deviation
C Central cyanosis
D Normal PaO_2 with reduced $PaCO_2$
E Reduced FVC
F Crepitations in the lower and mid zones

158. Which of the following are true:

A Radioisotope perfusion lung scanning can distinguish embolism from infection
B Lung scanning is a useful technique in the diagnosis of pulmonary embolism
C Asbestosis predisposes to mesothelioma formation
D Farmer's lung is a precipitin mediated reaction
E Linear atelectasis is a feature of pulmonary embolism and systemic lupus erythematosus
D Psittacosis is known as bird fancier's lung
G Paragonamiasis is known as bird fancier's lung

CARDIOVASCULAR DISEASE

159. Known risk factors in the development of ischaemic heart disease are:

A Diabetes mellitus
B Cigarette smoking
C Type IV hyperlipidaemia
D Heredity
E Hypertension

160. Following myocardial infarction:

A The immediate mortality from sudden death is about 25%

B Overall mortality is reduced if anticoagulants are given

C Dopamine may reverse the hypotension of shock

D Lignocaine is the treatment of choice for atrial ectopics

E Wenckebach phenomenon is diagnosed by finding a prolonged PR interval on ECG

F A pansystolic apical murmur suggests papillary muscle dysfunction

G Cardiac aneurysm is suggested by persistent ST elevation

161. Dressler's post-myocardial infarction syndrome is characterised by:

A Smooth muscle antibodies

B Pericardial friction

C Onset within 48 hours after infarction

D Pleural effusion

E Rapid response to steroids

162. Which of the following exclude myocardial infarction:

A Normal ECG

B No rise in the SGOT

C Pain lasting less than 20 min

D No radiation to the neck

E No radiation to the arms

163. Which of the following statements are true:

A Atrial fibrillation causes an irregular ventricular rhythm

B Atrial flutter usually causes an irregular ventricular rhythm

C In heart block after infarction the prognosis is better with inferior infarction than anterior infarction

D Epilepsy may be the presenting feature of complete heart block

E The 3rd heart sound is heard just before the 1st sound

164. In patients with suspected rheumatic fever:

A *Streptococcus viridans* is often grown from nose or throat culture

B Erythema nodosum is a major diagnostic criterion

C Chorea is a major diagnostic criterion

D Joint pains tend to be migratory mainly in large joints and exquisitely tender

E Constrictive pericarditis is a recognised complication

F The PR interval is typically prolonged

165. The 'opening snap' of mitral stenosis:

A Denotes valve mobility

B Disappears if atrial fibrillation occurs

C Is usually best heard at the apex

D Replaces the third heart sound

E Is really a 'closing snap'

166. If mitral stenosis is present in a pregnant woman she:

A Is in greatest danger in the 2nd trimester
B Should be delivered by Caesarian section
C May be symptom free after delivery
D Should be anticoagulated to prevent venous thrombosis and pulmonary embolism
E Will require prophylactic digoxin and diuretics before the 2nd trimester

167. Mitral regurgitation is associated with:

A Marfan's syndrome
B Ankylosing spondylitis
C Hypertensive heart disease
D Cardiomyopathy
E Thyrotoxicosis
F Myocardial infarction
G Syphylitic carditis

168. Which of the following are true of the effect of maternal rubella on the fetus:

A It is most dangerous in the 2nd trimester
B It may cause ASD, VSD or patent ductus arteriosus
C It may cause cerebellar degeneration
D It may cause deafness
E It may cause talipes equino-varus

169. In aortic stenosis:

A There is often a previous history of syphilis
B Fainting attacks may occur
C Sudden death may occur
D Angina is a common symptom
E A cardiac thrill is uncommon
F The second sound is quiet

170. An ostium-primum atrial septal defect:

A Is more common than an ostium secundum defect
B May be associated with a VSD
C Produces right axis deviation
D Produces left axis deviation
E The main QRS axis is normal
F Is more likely to become infected

171. Which of the following are recognised associations of a ventricular septal defect:

A Atrial fibrillation
B Infective endocarditis
C Mongolism
D Collapsing pulse
E Wide fixed splitting of the second sound

172. Fallot's tetralogy:

A Is the most common congenital heart disorder
B May present with syncope and squatting
C Is complicated by cerebral abscess formation
D Is associated with paradoxical emboli
E Is not always associated with cyanosis in the neonate

173. Diagnosis of infective endocarditis is supported by:

A Microscopic haematuria
B Rose spots
C Reduced complement levels
D Antigen–antibody complexes in the serum
E Culture of β-haemolytic streptococci from the throat
F Osler's nodes
G Conjunctival oedema

174. Pericarditis may be a feature of:

A Uraemia
B Coxsackie B infection
C Herpes simplex infection
D Systemic lupus erythematosus
E Myocardial infarction
F Bronchial carcinoma

175. In constrictive pericarditis:

A Orthopnoea occurs early in the disease
B Ascites occurs after ankle oedema
C Fatigue is an early feature
D Cannon waves are present in the JVP
E Pericardial friction rub is often present
F Calcification is not always present on the PA chest film but may be seen on the lateral X-ray

176. Uncontrolled hypertension increases the risk of:

A Early death
B Diabetes mellitus
C Myocardial infarction
D Pulmonary embolism
E Subdural haemorrhage
F Confusional state

177. All patients with hypertension require:

A An IVP
B An MSU
C An ECG
D A CXR
E A 24 hour urine protein estimation
F A VMA estimation
G An estimation of cortisol diurnal variation

178. Which of the following are true:

A Rib notching is seen on the upper rib border in aortic coarctation

B Diazoxide by mouth or injection is used to control malignant (accelerated) hypertension

C Accelerated hypertension is diagnosed by the occurrence of rapidly progressive cardiac failure

D Hydrallazine acts mainly on the vasomotor centre

E Reserpine acts mainly on the vasomotor centre

F Hypokalaemia and alkalosis in hypertension suggest Cushing's or Conn's syndrome

179. Intermittent claudication:

A Is associated with reduced life expectancy

B Is relieved by a α-receptor blocking agents

C Is improved by graded walking exercises

D Occurs in association with types III and IV hyperlipidaemia

180. Which of the following are associated with Raynaud's phenomenon:

A Colour changes in the order of white, red and blue

B Phaeochromocytoma

C Carcinoid syndrome

D Methyldopa

E Levodopa

F Scleroderma

G Chagas' disease

H Vibrating tools

181. The following are characteristic of psoriasis:
A Silver scales
B Wickham's striae
C Koebner's phenomenon
D Mucosal lesions
E Pruritus

182. The following characterise lichen planus:
A Silver scales
B Wickham's striae
C Koebner's phenomenon
D Mucosal lesions
E Pruritis

183. Which of the following are associated with arthritis:
A Pityriasis rosea
B Erythema marginatum
C Keratoderma blenorrhagica
D Lichen planus
E Psoriasis

184. Candidiasis may complicate:
A Diabetes mellitus
B Diabetes insipidus
C Hypoparathyroidism
D Pseudohypoparathyroidism
E Hyperthyroidism
F Hodgkin's disease

185. Erythema nodosum occurs with:

A Leprosy
B Schistosomiasis
C Toxoplasmosis
D Lincomycin therapy
E Gentamicin therapy
F Rheumatic fever
G Sarcoid

186. Lesions around the mouth are characteristically seen in:

A Sarcoidosis
B Dermatomyositis
C Hereditary haemorrhagic telangiectasia
D Crigler-Najjar syndrome
E Peutz-Jegher syndrome
F Herpes simplex infection

187. Mucosal ulceration occurs in:

A Infection with Coxsackie B virus
B Pernicious anaemia
C Behçet's syndrome
D Chickenpox
E Acute lymphatic leukaemia
F Pemphigus vulgaris

188. In pemphigoid:

A Mucosal ulceration is common
B Nikolski's sign is positive
C Underlying carcinoma may be present
D Prognosis is very poor
E Prednisolone may control the skin eruption

189. Which of the following commonly cause iron deficiency anaemia:

A Thalassaemia major
B Sickle cell anaemia
C Menorrhagia
D Ankylostoma duodenale
E Ascaris lumbricoides

190. Macrocytic anaemia is associated with:

A MCV of 80–86 fl
B MCV of 86–96 fl
C MCV of 96–106 fl
D Folic acid deficiency
E Chronic liver disease
F Chronic renal disease
G Primidone therapy

191. Megaloblasts:

A Are present in large numbers in the marrow in B_{12} deficiency
B Are normally present in insignificant numbers in the marrow
C Have polychromatic multilobed nuclei
D Are associated with leucopenia and thrombocytopenia

192. Pernicious anaemia is associated with:

A Antibodies to parietal cells
B Antibodies to intrinsic factor
C Antibodies to thyroid cytoplasm
D Antibodies to mitochondria
E Antibodies to smooth muscle

193. The following features occur in thrombotic thrombocytopenic purpura:

A Haemolytic anaemia and hyperbilirubinaemia
B Capillary and arteriolar thrombi in the kidneys
C Abnormal neurological signs
D LE cells in the peripheral blood
E Response to heparin

194. Paroxysmal nocturnal haemoglobinuria is associated with:

A Macrocytosis in the peripheral blood
B Chronic bronchitis and high PaO_2
C Positive Ham's test
D Reduced red cell acetyl cholinesterase
E Red cells in urine

195. In iron deficiency anaemia:

A The MCV is usually normal
B The MCH is usually reduced
C Plasma iron is less than 40μ mol/litre
D Iron binding capacity is above 65μ mol/litre

196. Eosinophilia in the peripheral blood is seen in:

A Polyarteritis nodosa
B Pulmonary aspergillosis
C Asthma
D Pulmonary sarcoidosis
E Interstitial pulmonary fibrosis

197. In polycythaemia rubra vera:

A Splenomegaly and lymphadenopathy are common
B The PaO_2 is usually reduced
C Central cyanosis may occur
D Red cell mass is increased
E WBC and platelet counts are raised

198. The bleeding time is prolonged in:

A Scurvy
B Secondary thrombocytopenia
C Haemophilia
D Christmas disease
E Osler Rendu Weber disease
F Osgood-Schlatter's disease
G von Willebrand's disease

199. Multiple myeloma is characterised by:

A Aplastic anaemia
B Hypercalcaemia
C Excess immunoglobulin, usually IgA
D Bence-Jones heavy chain immunoglobulins
E Raised plasma alkaline phosphatase

200. Generalised lymphadenopathy is characteristic of the following infections:

A Bacillary dysentery
B Schistosomiasis
C Toxoplasmosis
D Echinococcus
E Tuberculosis
F Recurrent malaria

201. In Hodgkin's disease:

- **A** Herpes zoster is common in untreated patients
- **B** Stage III indicates involvement above and below the diaphragm
- **C** The central nervous system is occasionally involved
- **D** Prognosis is better if the glands are lymphocyte free
- **E** Prognosis is better in men
- **F** 5-year survival with modern therapy is about 80%

202. Hereditary spherocytosis:

- **A** Is transmitted as an autosomal recessive
- **B** Produces unconjugated bilirubin in the urine
- **C** Is a rare cause of haemolytic crisis
- **D** Is prevalent because it protects against malaria
- **E** May present with cholecystitis

203. Leukaemia:

- **A** Total white cell count may be normal in acute lymphocytic leukaemia
- **B** Splenomegaly is a common presenting feature of acute lymphocytic leukaemia
- **C** The presence of Philadelphia chromosome is pathognomonic of chronic lymphocytic leukaemia
- **D** The Philadelphia chromosome is an abnormality of chromosome No. 23
- **E** In acute myeloid leukaemia, cranial irradiation is part of the standard regime

204. Which of the following compounds are dialysable:

A Benzodiazepines
B Tricyclic antidepressants
C Lithium
D Ferrous sulphate
E Paraquat
F Sodium salicylate

205. Specific antidotes exist for which of the following poisons:

A Paraquat
B Buprenorphine
C Paracetamol
D Benzodiazepines
E Tricyclic antidepressants

206. In paraquat poisoning:

A An airway must be stabilised early
B Bentonite should be given by slow i.v. infusion
C Emetics should be used
D Death always occurs without treatment
E Early dialysis is indicated

207. Typhoid:

A Classically begins with dry cough and constipation
B Is excluded by a normal WBC count
C Typically produces Roth spots on the lower chest, upper abdomen and flanks
D May cause intestinal perforation
E Chloramphenicol is the drug of first choice
F Responds also to ampicillin, metronidazole and co-trimoxazole

208. Falciparum malaria:

A Is also known as benign tertian malaria
B In Africa is often chloroquine resistant
C Can cause an acute confusional state
D Should be treated with primaquine to destroy the intrahepatic phase
E Does not cause acute haemolysis

CASE STUDIES

CASE 1

A 66-year old woman presents with lethargy, fatigue and dyspnoea on effort. She had a well-maintained appetite and had not lost weight. She had had no pain. Physical examination was within normal limits.

On investigation, routine haematology gave the following findings: Hb, 8·2 g/dl; PCV, 26; MCV, 76 fl; MCH, 24 pg; MCHC, 29 g/dl; ESR, 21 mm/h; retics, 3%.

a What kind of anaemia is this?
b What further direct questions do you wish to ask her?
c What further investigations would you perform?
d Which of the following, given your present information, might you perform as part of your immediate management: oral iron, parenteral iron; whole blood transfusion; B_{12} injections and/or oral folic acid; cimetidine?

CASE 2

A 40-year old woman is admitted to hospital with a 5 day history of the symptoms of a urinary tract infection and pain in the right loin and over the bladder. She has had a rigor and is now semi-conscious, disorientated and aggressive. On clinical examination, she was dehydrated and hyperventilating but there were no focal signs and no evidence of heart failure. There was no past history of respiratory disease.

a What is the likeliest diagnosis of the underlying disease?
b What investigations do you think are the most important in the initial investigation of this patient?
c List the 6 key points you must consider in the management of this patient

CASE 3

A 50-year old man was readmitted to hospital following a fourth episode in two years of loss of consciousness and aggressive confusion. There is no history of fits and no focal neurological lesion was described or cardiac dysrhythmia noted. He was cold and clammy initially but recovered spontaneously still showing no neurological signs. The skin was unusually smooth and he had only a light thin growth of body hair. His testicles were noted to be small.

a What was the immediate cause of his admission to hospital?
b What is this due to in his case?
c How would you set about confirming it clinically
 i using 3 main points from the history
 ii using 3 main signs on examination
 iii what investigations would you perform?

CASE 4

A 37-year old unemployed medical educationalist gives a 3 week history of intermittent shortness of breath and wheezing. He has just returned from a short stay in Nigeria. He has never smoked. On examination it is noticed that he is highly stressed. He was markedly dyspnoeic at rest and there was a generalised expiratory wheeze. There was no clubbing or cyanosis and no cardiac abnormality. Investigations were reported as follows: Hb, electrolytes, CXR and liver function tests all normal; WBC, 8200 with 10% eosinophils; ESR, 30 mm in 1 hour, blood urea 10 mmol/litre (60 mg/dl). Clinically he has asthma of late onset.

a What might spirometry show before and after bronchodilators?

b Give the important underlying disorders.

c How would you investigate him further in the first instance? Give 4 tests.

d How would you manage the presenting problem?

CASE 5

A 70-year old farmworker presents as an emergency after waking with a cold, painful and numb right leg from the mid-thigh downwards. No movements are present below the knee. On examination the limb is cold, pale, numb, cyanosed and immobile. The pulse is 120/min and in sinus rhythm, and the blood pressure 100 mmHg systolic (the diastolic is unrecordable).

a What is the clinical diagnosis?

b What are the possible underlying causes?

c Enumerate 6 possible factors which may be considered in the immediate management of this patient and discuss their relative importance.

d The leg improves spontaneously in the next few hours. What would be your further management of this patient if his general health also improved at the same time?

CASE 6A

A 60-year old Administrative Medical Officer was noticed by his colleagues to be slowing up more than expected (for his age) and especially so in the last 9 months. A medical opinion was sought. He walked slowly into the clinic and appeared apathetic and unresponsive. There were no specific features in the history.

a What initial diagnoses run through your mind?
b How would you investigate him initially? Suggest 2 tests.
c What should you tell the Senior Administrative Medical Officer about this?

CASE 6B

A similar patient was not depressed but treatment with levodopa produced dramatic improvement. Patients with Parkinsonism can present without observable tremor and the diagnosis is easily missed unless it is kept in mind in the differential diagnosis of the 'inert' patient. Such patients often respond well to modern therapy.

d How does the addition of a dopa decarboxylase inhibitor to levodopa affect its efficacy?
e What other treatments are available for the treatment of Parkinsonism?

CASE 7

A 65-year old postman was admitted for treatment to a large painful varicose leg ulcer which had failed to heal with conventional treatment over the last 2 years and from which β- haemolytic streptoccocci has been isolated. The infection was first treated with oral sulphadimidine and finally responded to a course of penicillin G and the ulcer healed over the course of the next 3 weeks. Just before discharge the House Physician noticed that the patient appeared cyanosed. The patient did not feel short of breath and there was no history of chest trouble. There were no abnormal physical signs in the chest and the CXR appeared normal. He had never been a smoker.

a What do you feel is the most likely diagnosis and what other conditions would you consider?

b How would you investigate him?

c If you think treatment is indicated, what would you use, and how long would you continue it?

CASE 8

A 27-year old girl came to the clinic with a 2 month history of progressive weakness during which she had noticed that she was able to get on her bicycle to go to work but unable to get off it easily. Recently her jaw had tended to stay open towards the end of a conversation. On examination she had mild bilateral ptosis and held her jaw closed with the left hand whilst giving the later part of her history.

a What diagnoses have run through your mind in a rough order of probability?

b Name one investigation which can be performed in the clinic and which may give an immediate diagnosis.

c If positive, what drug treatment might you use in her initial treatment?

d Give four main differences between your diagnosis and the Eaton-Lambert syndrome.

CASE 9

A 23-year old previously fit amateur footballer went to bed early telling his wife that he thought he was getting 'flu'. She watched television late and when she got to bed found him to be confused and disorientated. The general practitioner who called half an hour later, found him stuporose, diagnosed acute meningitis, and admitted him forthwith to hospital. On admission apart from the reduced level of consciousness, the only abnormal sign was severe neck stiffness. Lumbar puncture was performed and the CSF was reported as showing a protein concentration of 200 mg/dl (20 g/litre, 240 polymorphs and 20 lymphocytes and a Gram stain film showed Gram-positive intracellular diplococci.

a What is the responsible organism?

b Should antibacterial chemotherapy be started before the results of bacterial culture are available?

c What is your initial treatment of choice? What would you suggest as best second-line therapy? Give appropriate doses, frequency and route.

CASE 10

A 43-year old man, a known hypertensive, presents with jaundice. The liver function tests show a bilirubin (total) of 19 mmol/litre (11 mg/dl), an alkaline phosphatase of 92 IU/litre (upper limit of normal range; 90), an APT (SGPT) of 31 (upper limit normal; 32) and urine which contained urobilingen. The blood count showed a haemoglobin of 9 g/dl and the film was normocytic and normochromic. The reticulocyte count was 7%.

a What kind of anaemia is this?

b What are the commoner causes of it and which are the likeliest in this man?

c What investigations would help to confirm your provisional diagnosis?

CASE 11

A 23-year old man presents with a two month history of nocturnal fever, lassitude and weight loss. On examination, he is found to have pallor and enlarged lymph nodes on the left side of his neck. The spleen was just palpable. Lymph node biopsy was reported as follows: Many Reed-Sternberg cells present with plentiful lymphocytes; There is no fibrosis.

a What is your diagnosis?
b What features given above will guide your prognosis?
c What features given above will guide your therapy?

CASE 12

A 50-year old patient previously fit, presented with a 'flu'-like illness for two days, followed by jaundice on the third day which had persisted for the next fortnight. He had noticed that his urine had appeared dark and his stools pale. On examination his liver was just palpable but not tender. The liver function tests showed a moderately raised serum bilirubin and alkaline phosphatase and an SGPT (APT) about 3 times the upper limit of the normal range.

a What abnormalities do you expect to find in the urine on standard ward testing?
b What are the 4 most likely diagnoses in order of probability given the above facts?
c What further investigations would you perform?

ANSWERS

PART ONE

Question	*Answer*	*Question*	*Answer*	*Question*	*Answer*
1	BDE	16	BDE	31	BDE
2	ACD	17	ACEG	32	ABCF
3	AD	18	CD	33	BCE
4	ABD	19	D	34	AE
5	BCE	20	AD	35	ADEF
6	AD	21	ABEF	36	DEF
7	CD	22	CF	37	B
8	BCDF	23	ABCDEF	38	ACD
9	BE	24	AC	39	CD
10	CDE	25	ABDEF	40	AD
11	ACDEF	26	BCDE	41	BCD
12	BE	27	ACDF	42	ABD
13	C	28	BDE	43	BC
14	ABE	29	ACEF	44	ABCFG
15	ABDEF	30	ACD		

PART TWO

Question	*Answer*	*Question*	*Answer*	*Question*	*Answer*
45	CE	77	BDE	109	B
46	DE	78	CDF	110	DE
47	ABE	79	ABF	111	ABCDE
48	A	80	BCE	112	ABCDG
49	ABCDEF	81	BCDE	113	BCEG
50	ABCE	82	BCDE	114	ACDF
51	—	83	CE	115	BCE
52	AE	84	ABD	116	BD
53	ACDE	85	ACDE	117	BC
54	ABCDG	86	ABDE	118	CD
55	ABCDEFGH	87	BE	119	BCE
56	ABE	88	BD	120	B
57	CEF	89	BDE	121	CD
58	BDE	90	ADE	122	AC
59	CD	91	ABE	123	AE
60	AC	92	CD	124	C
61	—	93	BEG	125	ABD
62	ABD	94	ADE	126	B
63	ACD	95	BD	127	DF
64	ABE	96	CE	128	ACE
65	BCE	97	ABCD	129	B
66	CE	98	ABE	130	BD
67	BC	99	ACDE	131	ACDE
68	ABCDE	100	CD	132	ABDF
69	ACDEF	101	ACDEF	133	ABCD
70	ACD	102	ABCDE	134	BCEF
71	ADE	103	ACD	135	BE
72	BDE	104	CD	136	AD
73	ABD	105	BCE	137	BC
74	—	106	AD	138	BDEG
75	ABCDE	107	AC	139	ABEG
76	BCD	108	CD	140	E

Question	*Answer*	*Question*	*Answer*	*Question*	*Answer*
141	ABCD	164	CDF	187	CDEF
142	AE	165	A	188	CE
143	ABD	166	C	189	CD
144	ACEF	167	ABCDF	190	CDEG
145	CDGH	168	BD	191	AD
146	AB	169	BCDF	192	ABC
147	BDE	170	BDF	193	ABCDE
148	AC	171	BC	194	ACD
149	BCDEG	172	BCDE	195	BCD
150	BD	173	ACDF	196	ABC
151	ABCD	174	ABDEF	197	CDE
152	AEF	175	CF	198	ABG
153	BE	176	ACF	199	AB
154	ADE	177	BCD	200	CE
155	AB	178	EF	201	BCF
156	CF	179	ACD	202	CE
157	ACEF	180	FH	203	A
158	BCDE	181	A	204	CEF
159	ABCDE	182	BCDE	205	BC
160	ACFG	183	BCE	206	CE
161	BDE	184	ACDF	207	ADE
162	—	185	ACFG	208	C
163	ACD	186	CEF		

ANSWERS TO CASE STUDIES

CASE 1

a 'Iron deficiency anaemia'

b Enquire about (i) any bleeding anywhere particularly from gut or vagina; (ii) drugs, especially analgesics; (iii) indigestion; (iv) change in bowel habit. Enquire about diet particularly in the elderly.

c Faeces for occult blood. Serum iron and total iron binding capacity. Sigmoidoscopy. If the results confirm the diagnosis of iron deficiency and there are not localising symptoms or signs, proceed to barium enema. If normal, proceed to barium swallow and meal.

d Oral iron

CASE 2

a Diabetes mellitus

b Blood sugar. Blood urea and electrolytes. Urine for microscopy and bacteriology. Routine haematology including white cell differential. Arterial blood for acid–base status. Blood culture.

c Fluid balance. Method and dose of insulin. Diagnosis and treatment of urinary tract infection. Serum potassium concentration and potassium balance. Aspiration of stomach. Acid–base status.

CASE 3

a Hypoglycaemia, possibly with hypoadrenalism.
b Pituitary failure.
c i Aggression is characteristic of hypoglycaemia. Reduced frequency of shaving. An increased tendency to feel the cold.
ii The skin is fine and hairless. Look for bitemporal hemianopia. Small testicles.
iii Serum cortisol with diurnal variation. Cortisol production rate. Serum thyroxine and TSH. Serum FSH/LH. Synacthen (tetracosactrin) test. X-ray the pituitary fossa.

NB Treatment should include parenteral cortisol (hydrocortisone) as well as glucose.

CASE 4

a A grossly reduced FEV1 (if he is capable of performing the test at all) e.g., 0·5–1·0 litre in one second. The FVC is commonly much reduced and the vital capacity usually cannot be fully expelled because of the airways obstruction. After bronchodilators, there is usually considerable improvement toward normal.
b Pulmonary eosinophilia due to filariasis. Polyarteritis nodosa. Extrinsic allergic alveolitis. Aspergillosis.
c Urine for red cells. Stools for cysts, ova, worms. IVP and consider renal biopsy if PN is a reasonable possibility.
Testing of skin or bronchial hypersensitivity is unlikely to be helpful. (Chest X-ray has already been performed.)
d Intravenous hydrocortisone, B_2-agonist (e.g., salbutamol, terbutaline), aminophylline and fluids. High concentration oxygen (e.g., 40–50%). Antifilarial therapy may be necessary.

CASE 5

a Acute obstruction of the femoral artery.
b Embolism possibly from the left atrium with paroxysmal atrial fibrillation, and thrombosis.
c Keep the limb cool. Consider surgical disobliteration. Rest. Give oxygen in high concentration (possibly hyperbaric if available). Anticoagulate (with heparin by infusion and followed by oral anticoagulants). Infuse low molecular weight dextrans. Thrombolytic agents. Vasodilators.
d Continue conservative medical management. Mobilise early. Discharge as soon as possible if the limb remains viable and preferably off all treatment.

CASE 6A

a Depression. Presenile dementia. Hypothyroidism. Parkinsonism. Sedative drug abuse.
b Thyroid function tests. Serum barbiturate.
c Nothing.

CASE 6B

d The addition of a dopa decarboxylase inhibitor tends to prevent the breakdown of administered levodopa to dopamine in the peripheral tissues and there is thus a reduction in the side effects due to the peripheral actions of levodopa metabolites (especially nausea and vomiting and to a lesser extent hypotension). The dose of levodopa is much reduced to obtain the same effect on the Parkinsonism.
e Anticholinergic drugs. Amantidine. Bromocryptine. Physiotherapy. Stereotactic surgery. Antidepressant drugs (excluding MAOI drugs) if necessary.

CASE 7

a Multiple pulmonary emboli is the most likely diagnosis. Polycythaemia rubra vera may be associated with leg ulcers. Methaemoglobinaemia may result from some sulphonamides and primaquine therapy.

b Recheck the CXR for attenuation of peripheral vessels — easily missed. Lung perfusion scan. Haemoglobin and PVC. Arterial blood gases of PaO_2. Blood spectroscopy for methaemoglobin.

c Heparin initially and warfarin for 3 months. Polycythaemia rubra vera may require venesection; chemotherapy may also be used. Lifelong follow up is necessary. No treatment is required for methaemoglobinaemia in the absence of symptoms other than the removal of an identified cause; spontaneous recovery is the rule.

CASE 8

a Myasthenia gravis, hysteria, familial periodic paralysis, facio-scapular-humeral muscular dystrophy, Eaton-Lambert syndrome, hypokalaemia.

b Intravenous edrophonium (Tensilon) 10 mg should result in an immediate and dramatic reduction in muscular weakness in patients with myasthenia gravis.

c Pyridostigmine. Between 5 and 20 tablets (60 mg) may be required in one day divided into several doses per day (i.e. 300–1200 mg daily dose). Initial doses should be small and the dose gradually worked up. Overdose may give depolarisation block with weakness. An alternative is neostigmine one or two 15 mg tablets at a time. They need to be given more frequently than pyridostigmine because of their shorter duration of action.

d In the Eaton-Lambert syndrome the facial muscles are less affected than the limb muscles (especially the proximal muscles); muscle strength may initially be increased by repeated movements; there is no response to edrophonium; a carcinoma frequently of the bronchus, is usually identifiable.

CASE 9

a Pneumococcal meningitis. Acute meningitis.
b Yes. Even brief delay in starting effective therapy can result in increased morbidity and mortality.
c Benzyl-penicillin 12–20 megaunits intravenously per 24 hours in divided doses (6-hourly). Chloramphenicol 1 g 6-hourly initially.

CASE 10

a Intrinsic red cell disorders e.g. haemoglobinopathies, G6PD deficiency, hereditary spherocytosis.
b Autoimmune acquired. Idiopathic or drugs.
c Direct Coomb's test is positive in haemolytic jaundice due to autoimmune disease and methyldopa therapy.

CASE 11

a Hodgkin's disease, clinically Stage IIIB.
b Though the lymphadenopathy is clinically confined to one region, the presence of a palpable spleen stages his disease as not less than Stage III.
The presence of plentiful lymphocytes is a good prognostic feature.
c The staging of Hodkin's disease determines therapy as well as prognosis. Patients with the staging of IIIB are now customarily treated with multiple chemotherapy and radiotherapy.

CASE 12

a The presence of bilirubin and urobilin in excess.

b Carcinoma of the head of the pancreas, obstruction of the bile duct by a gall stone, drug jaundice, infectious hepatitis.

c None of the history strongly suggests drug jaundice. If jaundice improves, infectious hepatitis, drugs or gall stones become likely and cholangiography should be performed to exclude stones. If obstructive jaundice persists, proceed to ultrasound and liver scan (to detect enlarged ducts), percutaneous cholangiography with arrangements to proceed to liver biopsy or laparotomy if necessary.